Starch solution cookbook for starters

Change your life eat the food you love lose weight and overcome food addiction

By

David Pish

Table of contents

There are several vegan diet options, but high-carb, low-fat has become more and more popular in the past ten years.

contends that consuming whole-food, plant-based carbohydrates can actually aid in weight loss, despite the widespread belief among specialists that eating carbohydrates causes weight gain (thus the popularity of the ultra-low-carb keto diet).

What Exactly Is a Starch Solution?

The Starch Solution is a high-carb, low-fat vegan diet with a focus on eating entire, plant-based foods, no oil, no processed food, and little to no sugar.

You avoid all animal products and concentrate your meals on starchy foods like whole grains, potatoes, vegetables, and fruits.

the advantages of a whole-food, plant-based, high-starch diet, including how it may give you energy, sate your appetite,and help you maintain a healthy weight.

Additionally, the book describes how this diet can guard against long-term illnesses like high cholesterol, heart disease, acne, and type 2 diabetes.

The fact that you can still eat foods like bread, pasta, burritos, pizza, pancakes, and ice cream while adhering to the Starch Solution makes it so accessible to everyone.

especially those coming from the Standard American Diet (SAD), which is high in meat, dairy, and highly-processed, nutrient-poor foods.

Simply consume wholesome, plant-based alternatives.

Continue reading to find out which meals to prioritize, which are forbidden, which plant-based foods to stay away from if your weight loss has plateaued,and what the experts say of the Starch Solution.

What Foods on the Starch Solution Should You Avoid?

Meat including fish, poultry, beef, and pork.
Eggs.

milk, cheese, yogurt, ice cream, and butter, among other dairy items
Oil, such as canola, coconut, avocado, and olive oil.

packaged and processed foods.

What Meals Are Recommended While Using the Starch Solution?

Oats, brown rice, quinoa, barley, millet, farro, corn, rye, spelt, and wheat berries are examples of starchy whole grains.

Whole grain products such as bread, cereals, pasta, couscous, tortillas, and flatbreads are available.

Lentils, peas, such as green peas, split peas, and black-eyed peas, as well as all dried legumes, such as kidney, black, navy, adzuki, cannellini, garbanzo, pinto, and soybeans.

starchy vegetables, such as potatoes and sweet potatoes, corn, winter squashes like spaghetti and butternut.

Greens, broccoli, cauliflower, cabbage, asparagus, brussels sprouts, carrots, cucumbers, zucchini, yellow squash, bell peppers, tomatoes, celery, onions, mushrooms, radishes, snap peas, snow peas, green beans, and eggplant are examples of non-starchy vegetables. Fruits such as berries, citrus, apples, bananas, melons, mangoes, kiwis, peaches, pineapple, and grapes, both fresh and frozen.

little amounts of sweets, such as a dash of maple syrup on your whole wheat pancakes, a sprinkle of brown sugar on your oatmeal, or a dollop of ketchup with your oil-free, oven-baked fries
spices and herbs.

Use salt sparingly; instead of incorporating it into meals while they are being prepared, sprinkle a little on top of your plate or bowl.

What Foods on the Starch Solution Should You Avoid?

The following foods are permitted on the Starch Solution, although if weight loss is your aim, these foods will "slow your progress." So if your weight reduction has stopped, he advised, "I recommend avoiding these foods," and you can reintroduce them once you accomplish your target.

On the other hand, it's acceptable to include tiny amounts of these higher-calorie foods with your starch-based meals if you're content with your weight or aren't in a rush to reduce it.

Nuts such as almonds, walnuts, cashews, and peanuts, as well as nut butters prepared from them, and seeds including flax, chia, sesame, and sunflower
Fruits high in fat, such as avocado, olives, and coconut.

Dates, cranberries, and other dried fruits
Whole grain, wheat, and all-purpose flours
fresh fruit or vegetable juices.

White or brown sugar, coconut sugar, maple syrup, molasses, or agave nectar are examples of simple sugars.

Will Eating Foods High in Starch Make Me Gain Weight?

Just to be clear, the Starch Solution emphasizes consuming whole-food, plant-based meals instead of.

highly-processed,and high-fat starches for example cookies, cakes, french fries, including potato chips.

These foods include brown rice, oats, potatoes, beans, and fruit.

It's a frequent misperception that consuming starchy meals will result in weight gain.

"Starchy foods would not make you gain weight.

Because they are unprocessed, packed with water, and high in fiber, whole meals like these actually help you feel fuller for longer.

Although potatoes are a terrific example of a starchy carbohydrate that keeps you full and content.

Because of the way we prepare them, potatoes have a negative reputation and are seen as unhealthy.

For instance, we enjoy making potato chips or fries by frying them in oil, or we top baked potatoes with butter, sour cream, cheese, and bacon.

In order to make mashed potatoes, individuals typically use heavy cream and butter.

Your starchy, high-carb recipes may be so calorie-dense because of the additional fat, which you then link to weight gain.

Keep in mind that our body uses carbohydrates as its primary source of energy.

We should get about half of our calories from carbohydrates.

Getting out carbs from whole foods like fruits, vegetables, legumes, grains, and beans rather than meals with added sugar like cookies, cakes, pastries, drinks, and candies is more nutrient-dense and satiating.

How Can Enough Protein Be Added to the Starch Solution?

How Can Enough Protein Be Added to the Starch Solution?

There is a ton of protein in plants, particularly in beans, lentils, whole grains, and leafy greens.

If you consume enough calories from these foods, you will easily meet your protein goal.

Eight grams of protein can be found in a typical serving of whole wheat pasta, which is Starch-Solution-approved.

You might not need as much protein as you believe, the majority of Americans consume more protein than is essential.

spotting a person lacking in protein is quite uncommon.

"You can get plenty of protein in a balanced diet, even if you tend to be a vegan.

For the average adult, 50 to 60 grams of protein per day are usually plenty, according to her.

Olive and coconut oils aren't necessarily healthy.

Olive and coconut oils aren't necessarily healthy.

If you consider how [oils are] produced, you will see that they are also processed foods."

Processing removes the water and the fiber from olives, avocados, peanuts, or coconuts, leaving only the pure fat.

Two tablespoons of peanut butter are 190 calories and one tablespoon of olive oil is 119 calories," she said, "oils are the highest calorie food there is per pound."

Eating plant-based, high-fat foods in their whole-food form is the best way to reap the nutritional benefits of healthy fats, which include antioxidants, vitamins, minerals, and fiber. Saint-Laurent.

monitoring your portion sizes by pointing out that plant lipids also help you feel full.

She added that, in contrast to other plant oils, which are unsaturated fats, coconut oil is a saturated fat and should only be.

consumed in moderate amounts due to its association with heart disease.

The Starch Solution Diet: Is It Safe Over Time?

The Starch Solution is fantastic since it can match anyone's demands,

who said she heartily recommends it to clients.

You'll feel incredibly satiated after eating a diet high in fiber and low in fat, and intuitive eating is simple.

You can obtain all of your needs from a high-carb, whole-food, plant-based diet.

The only two things I would add are to take vitamin D3 and a B12 pill.

always consult their doctors and dietitians before changing their diets.

As food plays a significant role in our social lives, it should promote joy rather than worry.

The ultimate goal of your diet should be to promote health and happiness, and any balanced diet that allows you to consume the foods that make you feel good and incorporates a wide variety of nutrients may be maintained over the long term. This method of eating is worth it.

experimenting to see if you like it.

A 2 WEEK STARCH SOLUTION DIET MEAL PLAN

I want to give you a meal plan that will make following the Starch Solution Diet easier.

Breakfast, lunch, plus dinner are all included in this.

I also have a list of snacks at the conclusion.

Meal planning suggestions are also included in this starch solution menu for each week.

If you have children at home, this meal plan is perfect because everyone can eat the same meals.

Always include cooked/steamed non-starchy vegetables or an additional half-plate salad with your meal for best weight loss.

ARE CALORIE COUNTS REQUIRED?

The entire point of the Starch Solution Diet is to eliminate the necessity for calorie counting.

You consume a lot of whole grains, veggies, and both starchy and non starchy vegetables that are low in calories.

Oils, fat, cheese, sugar, and processed foods are all strictly prohibited as are other high-calorie items.

There are some nuts, seeds, and avocado in this meal plan, but not every day; you are free to exclude them if you like.

Week 1 of the Starch Solution diet food

Choose from these options for breakfast.

Almond porridge.

Rollin Oats, 70g. Consume with 1/2 cup berries.

Eat non-starchy vegetables like tomatoes, cucumbers, bell peppers, fried cabbage, or steamed broccoli if you're still hungry.

overnight oats cooked with fruit, berries, and plant milk.

Toast with vegetables and hummus.

1 baked tiny sweet potato.

Eat this dish salty with silken tofu mayo and beans or sweet with berries or other fruits.

Waffle iron-cooked hash browns prepared with shredded potatoes.

Green beans, tomatoes, bell peppers, or other vegetables with tofu scramble. smoothie mug.

Ideas for starchy meals for lunch and dinner…

Lunch and supper suggestions for the starch solution diet.

LUNCH DINNER MONDAY Pie with lentilsFries or oven slices of potatoes and salad.

TUESDAY steamed broccoli with boiled whole grain pasta with "cheese sauce"Pie with lentils.

WEDNESDAY Noodle saladBeans, rice, and fried broccoli.

THURSDAY salad with beans and riceSpanish rice

FRIDAY Remainings or a chickpea salad tacos de mussel.

SUNDAY Remaining tacos Pizza

SUNDAY Remaining pizza bean burger
Sunday night:

Get lots of potatoes ready! Make the shepherd's pie using lentils.

To have salad available for a few days, chop some up and put them in boxes. Construct the cheese sauce.

Make oil-free fries on Monday in the oven or air fryer and serve with ketchup or tofu mayo.

Add a half-plate of cooked non-starchy vegetables or a salad.

For Tuesday and Wednesday lunches, boil a bunch of whole-grain pasta along with some broccoli.

Tuesday: Prepare the spaghetti salad in advance for Wednesday's lunch.

Cook the double whole grain rice on Wednesday.

On a pan, cook some fried broccoli. Use canned beans for convenience (season with garlic, ginger, and soy sauce). Prepare the rice and bean salad for the next day.

Use the remaining rice to make the Mexican fried rice on Thursday.

Prepare the salad for lunch the next day.

It's taco day on Friday.

Pick a vegan taco recipe without oil, like mushroom tacos.

Make some pizza on Saturday and let each person pick their preferred toppings. I adore cherry tomatoes, roasted bell peppers, and arugula.

Make some bean burgers on Sunday. Roast some vegetables for Monday.
Week 2 of the Starch Solution diet.

A FEW MORE IDEAS FOR BREAKFAST

Eat cooked oats as a savory side dish with fried vegetables or with an apple or banana.

prepared quinoa.

Serve this dish savory with steamed or fried vegetables, or sweet with plant milk, cinnamon, cardamom, and shredded apple.

Banana-oat pancakes

Toast with scrambled tofu

Chia or linen seeds in a green smoothie
LUNCH DINNER.

MONDAY roasted vegetables in a salad Vegan bolognese over whole grain pasta or quinoa with roasted vegetables.

TUESDAY spaghetti and bolognese sweet potatoes baked with beans, salsa, and salad.

WEDNESDAY Kale and sweet potato salad stir-fried noodles with tofu.

THURSDAY leftover stir-fry noodlesRisotto
FRIDAY Remaining risotto

Lasagna SATURDAY leftover salad and lasagna curry with rice and greens
SUNDAY brunch with sandwiches or leftovers squash soup.

Monday: Make the vegan bolognese on Monday and cook some extra pasta or quinoa for the next day's lunch.

Tuesday: Baked sweet potatoes.

Prepare some extras for lunch that you can bake in cube form.

Wednesday: prepare a straightforward stir-fry with whole-grain rice noodles.

Make enough to last till lunch.

Choose a risotto dish for Thursday; I recommend lemon risotto.

Just omit the oil.

Make some delicious veggie lasagna on Friday; omit the vegan cheese and the extra virgin olive oil.

Rice and green curry on Saturday.

Instead of using oil, you can sauté the onions in vegetable broth.

The ordinary coconut milk can be substituted for the high-fat coconut milk.

Sunday: A sandwich breakfast can be a lovely weekend activity.

For instance, hollandaise sauce made without oil and whole-grain bread with tofu scramble.

To make this dish more full, add lentils or canned beans.

Make sure you bring any leftovers to work the following day.

FOOD IDEAS

Crispy kale

Sticks of carrot and hummus

You can substitute date paste or maple syrup for the sugar in chocolate pudding.

zero-fat vegan yogurt with fruit or berries
broccoli wings.

Sweet potato or potato chips cooked in the air.

- sweetened rice
- Oatmeal dates
- ice cream with bananas
- Salsa-topped nachos
- Sticks of cucumber with ranch dressing
- Popcorn made with air

YOU SHOULD EAT LIKE THIS TO ACHIEVE MAXIMUM WEIGHT LOSS

Consume 50/50 plates. So, always make some salad in addition to the main dishes, and only serve yourself half a plate of each.

With soup and salad, fill your stomach. Making this cabbage soup in addition to other meals is a terrific idea because it is so low in calories and gives you more vegetables and fiber.

One or two pieces of fruit maximum per day.

Learn about calorie density; reduce your intake of high-calorie items for a while, such as nuts, avocados, and products made with wheat, and replace them with more salads, soups, fruit, cooked starches like beans, potatoes, rice, and quinoa, as well as a small amount of non starchy vegetables.

less caloric.

Avoid eating in the late evening and aim to go a 12-hour night without eating to lose the most weight possible.

Non-starchy vegetables make excellent evening snacks.

I frequently get asked this question as a weight reduction coach. Am I still able to shed weight if I take smoothies for my breakfast?"

While it's true that you shouldn't eat calories via drinking if you want to lose weight, smoothies and soups should be the exception.I'll explain.

Juices are made by separating the fiber, which keeps you full and aids in weight loss, from the sugar and water and discarding the fiber.

Although mixing fruit significantly increases its calorie density, you are still eating the complete fruit when you drink smoothies.

just not in its entirety.

I personally advise my customers to drink smoothies, with one exception, as a delightful and practical method to ingest fruit and veggies.

Only when someone is only 5 to 10 pounds away from their weight reduction target and not losing any more weight would I advise decreasing smoothie consumption.

in recent weeks.

This most likely indicates that they have reached an equilibrium in their weight loss and that they need to slightly cut the calorie density of their meals in order to shed the final few pounds.

In this situation, making a few dietary adjustments, such as choosing whole fruit over smoothies, may help you lose the final few pounds.

A large handful of leafy greens can also offer a lot of nutritious value to your smoothie while lowering its calorie content.

I hope this makes it clearer why, for the most part, I don't advise skipping smoothies to lose weight.

The majority of people can lose weight when consuming a fruit and vegetable smoothie every day.

The Advantages Of A Diet High In Starches

Have you been interested in learning more about the benefits of a diet high in starches?

You're not by yourself, for sure.

Nowadays, more people are adopting healthier behaviors to enhance their physical well-being and encourage weight loss.

So it makes sense to investigate the potential effects of a low-starch diet on your general welfare.

Diet based on starch

What Exactly Is a High Starch Food Diet?

Only recently has the idea of a starch-based diet attracted a lot of attention, and this trend looks to be here to stay.

Sometimes, nutritional advice is just as fad-driven and fluid as fashion.

Other foods are the key to thriving good health and weight management,while others are deemed unhealthy and should be avoided.

The inverse seems to be true the next year.

Therefore, carbs become the nutritional evil to be avoided at all costs when highly meat-based, protein-driven diets like Atkins and Paleo reign supreme as a strategy to reduce weight.

But what if I told you that there are studies and other pieces of evidence that point to a starch-based diet as the one that has supported more people over the course of countless centuries?

To put it another way, during the vast majority of human history, the majority of people consumed staple diets of rice, potatoes, beans, corn, and sweet potatoes, along with various vegetables and seasonal fruit of course.

What kinds of starch-based foods ought to be a part of your diet? Now let's quickly review several beneficial carbohydrates for weight loss.

Cornmeal and Healthy Starches for Weight Loss.

Because it can be combined with so many other ingredients and has such a low saturated fat content, cornmeal is one of the greatest foods to include in a starch-based diet.

The most well-known source of starch is undoubtedly potatoes, which may be prepared in a variety of ways.

Additionally, potatoes are a great source of potassium, fiber, and B-complex vitamins.

Lentils

Additionally, foods containing resistant starch should be mentioned because they cannot be digested.

They will give you satiety feelings for longer lengths of time after eating, just like fiber does.

This group includes kidney beans, chickpeas, and baked beans.

In today's society, the expression "starch solution weight loss" has become a cliché. But some approaches are better than others.

Runner Eats Vegan

The 8 Best Tips for Cooking Without Oil

Today, I'd like to discuss oil-free cooking techniques and the many health benefits that may result from doing so for your vegan diet.

Using No Oil While Cooking: 8 Practical Tips.

You may wonder why we would want to cook without using any oil.

If you haven't noticed, one of the most divisive issues among vegan chefs and cookbook authors is whether to cook with or without oil.

According to one school of thinking, vegan butter, vegan margarine, vegan.

shortening, vegan oils of all kinds, etc., are worth utilizing in our kitchens as long as they are cruelty-free.

Another school of thought contends that regularly utilizing all of the aforementioned ingredients in your cooking will be harmful to your health, beginning with chronic inflammation (the root cause of numerous chronic diseases in the West) and possibly progressing to heart disease, diabetes, and even cancer.

Why Not Cook Without Oil?

Oil is a highly processed food with very few nutritional remnants.

The miraculous impact those "heart-healthy" olive and coconut oils will have on our wellbeing have been well-publicized.

However, the Nutrition Facts label on each bottle of oil reads, "Not a significant source of vitamin A, vitamin C, calcium, or iron" (which is present on most packaged foods in the US).

Few nutrients remain after the intensive filtration and refining process that produces the oil that we are familiar with and use.

Oil begins to become bad as soon as it is squeezed.

That's just how long-chain fatty acids, which are present in vegetable oils, live. Manufacturers put oils through a ton of processing and hydrogen atom addition to make them more shelf-stable and usable in high heat settings.

'Partially hydrogenated' may have appeared on the labels of several fatty foods.

What other by-product of hydrogenation is there? Trans fat. No matter the school of thinking we follow, those are useless to us.

Oil damages our arteries.

The endothelium (the inner lining) of our arteries is the entry point for cardiovascular disease.

But all hope is not lost.

Because our arterial lining has a propensity to heal itself, research has demonstrated that even the most severe cases of heart disease can be healed on a whole plant food, oil- and added fat-free diet.

Oil adds unwanted fat.

In actuality, the majority of the fat we eat is stored as body fat.

Only around 3% of the calories from fat are burnt during this shift, which plants fat where we least want it.

Mother Nature played a cruel trick on us by making this transition so simple.

It's interesting to note that a sample of a person's bodily fat tissue can reveal precisely which type of fat that person prefers.

People who consume a lot of junk food that contains margarine or shortening have high levels of trans fat in their body fat tissue, whereas people who enjoy.

cold-water marine seafood has higher levels of omega-3 fats in their soft tissues.

The fat we consume is the fat we wear.

We get as fat as we consume.

So what can we do to reduce the amount of oil we use in our regular cooking without sacrificing flavor?

8 Tips for Cooking Without Oil

1. When cooking food on the stovetop, use water or vegetable broth.

Add 1-2 Tbsp of water or broth to the heated pan or saucepan.

Follow your recipe as you normally would if you had started with oil until the liquid becomes frothy.

In order to keep the food from sticking to the pan, you might need to add more liquid.

I have never encountered a soup or stew recipe in my plant-based cooking practice that could not have been created using this technique with no oil.

Use a high-quality nonstick pan.

When preparing dishes without using oil, nonstick cookware can be quite helpful. The most popular cookware on the market is made of Teflon, but if you're worried about Teflon's potential health risks, consider ceramic-coated pots and pans. Amore Flamekiss cookware with a nano-ceramic covering is believed to be excellent.

3. When baking, use parchment paper.
Your meal won't stick to the pan as much using parchment paper.

This works best for baking tofu, vegan meatloaves, casseroles, brownies, quiches, etc. — anything that would ordinarily require pre-greasing the pan.

For instructions on baking oil-free tofu, read this post.

4. Substitute whole-food, plant-based ingredients for oils in baked goods.

Applesauce, bananas, ground flax, pureed legumes, non-dairy yogurt, etc. are excellent alternatives to baking items that include oil or other fats.

In my piece

How to Replace Butter and Eggs in Vegan Baking and Not End Up with Cardboard.

I went into great length about healthy vegan baking.

5. Use homemade salad dressings free of oil.

Keep checking back because I'll soon create a lengthy piece about my favorite quick and simple (you don't even need a blender!) oil-free salad dressings.

Please keep in mind that, until that time, a simple lime wedge squeezed over your salad can provide a ton of flavor without making you fat from processed fats.

See my post with 10 simple oil-free vegan salad dressing recipes, each of which takes less than two minutes to prepare, to get a better idea of how to make your own oil-free salad dressings.

Important nutrients may be better absorbed in salads with a small amount of fat, but it's always preferable to receive your fat from complete, unprocessed foods.

Add some diced avocado or a spoonful of raw pumpkin seeds to your salad as a garnish.

6. If necessary, use an oil mister or sprayer.

When toasting spices to enhance their flavor in Indian cuisine or roasting potatoes and other vegetables in the oven, a small amount of oil may be required in some circumstances.

An oil mister/sprayer like this one might be helpful in certain circumstances.

Spray a little oil in the center of the pan and toast your spices there, or drizzle a little oil over the vegetables before roasting.

7. The towel-paper trick

Do not desire to purchase an oil sprayer. add a few drops of oil to a heated skillet, spread it out, and then wipe part of it off with a paper towel as another way to reduce the amount of oil in your dish.

8. Look for recipes without oil.

If you start with recipes that are intended to be oil-free, cooking without oil will be much simpler.

See the recipe page for more information. The majority of the recipes on Vegan Runner Eats don't use any oil.

Is oatmeal a fiber or a starch?
For many years, oatmeal has been a favored breakfast food.

It is hearty, cozy, and warm.

Oatmeal is a complete grain and a good source of starch and fiber, so whether you eat it for breakfast or at any other time of the day, it adds nutrition to your balanced diet.

The Nutrition of Oats

Oatmeal is a fantastic source of a variety of nutrients your body needs for optimum health and is low in calories and high in fiber.

Oatmeal cooked in its natural state includes 170 calories per cup, 28 grams of carbohydrates, 6 grams of protein, and 4 grams of fiber.

It is also free of fat. The 1-cup portion also provides more than 10% of the daily requirements for thiamine, iron, zinc, and copper selenium and manganese.

Defined starch.

Starch is a kind of carbohydrate that is primarily present in some vegetables, such potatoes and corn, as well as in grains, like wheat, rice, and oats.

The starch in oatmeal gives your body energy because it is a carbohydrate.

Your body converts the starches in a bowl of whole-grain cereal into glucose, which gives your cells the energy they need to function.

It takes your body a little bit longer to break down starch because it is a complex carbohydrate as opposed to a simple carbohydrate like sugar.

advantages of oat fiber.

Soluble and insoluble fiber are the two main forms of fiber.

Soluble fiber slows down digestion in your digestive system, keeping you satisfied for a longer period of time.

When ingested, insoluble fiber improves stool quality and prevents constipation by acting more like a bulking agent.

Rich in soluble fiber is oatmeal.

This type of fiber not only prevents hunger pains but also lowers blood cholesterol levels and promotes heart health by grabbing onto cholesterol in the digestive tract and dragging it out of the body through the gel that is generated by the soluble fiber.

Oatmeal as a Part of Your Diet
On a chilly winter morning, nothing screams comfort quite like a hot dish of oats.

However, you do not need to stop eating oatmeal throughout the summer.

Serve the oatmeal cold the next morning for breakfast rather than heated by soaking the oats in milk or almond milk overnight with your preferred toppings.

Oats can also be added to your fruit and vegetable smoothie to thicken it and offer a bit more nutrition.

Additionally, you can use oatmeal in place of breadcrumbs in meatloaf.

Printed in Great Britain
by Amazon

26339948R00031